RETINOBLASTOMA

SIMPLE FACTS ABOUT CURING
RETINOBLASTOMA

DR. SARA WILLIAMS

Contents

CHAPTER ONE

DEFINITION

Retinoblastoma is an eye fixed most cancers that starts inside the retina the sensitive lining on the inside of your eye. Retinoblastoma most commonly affects younger children, however can not often occur in adults.

Your retina is made of nerve tissue that senses mild because it comes through the front of your eye. The retina sends alerts thru your optic nerve on your mind, where those indicators are interpreted as photographs.

A unprecedented form of eye most cancers, retinoblastoma is the most not unusual shape of cancer affecting the attention in kids. Retinoblastoma can also arise in one or both eyes.

Signs and symptoms of retinoblastoma encompass:

A white colour within the middle circle of the attention (student) whilst mild is shone in the eye, together with while taking a flash photograph

Eyes that appear like searching in specific instructions

Eye redness

Eye swelling

Whilst to see a medical doctor

Make an appointment together with your baby's health practitioner in case you observe any modifications in your child's eyes that concern you. Retinoblastoma is an extraordinary most cancers, so your baby's doctor may also discover other extra common eye situations first.

If you have a own family history of retinoblastoma, ask your pediatrician when your baby must start everyday eye assessments to display for retinoblastoma.

Causes

Retinoblastoma happens whilst nerve cells in the retina broaden genetic mutations. Those mutations purpose the cells to keep growing and multiplying whilst healthy cells would die. Retinoblastoma cells can invade in addition into the eye and close by systems. Retinoblastoma can also unfold (metastasize) to different areas of the frame, inclusive of the mind and backbone.

In the general public of instances, it's now not clean what reasons the genetic mutations that result in retinoblastoma. However, it is feasible for youngsters to inherit a genetic mutation from their parents.

Retinoblastoma this is inherited

Gene mutations that boom the chance of retinoblastoma and other cancers may be passed from dad and mom to youngsters. Hereditary retinoblastoma is handed from parents to children in an autosomal dominant sample, which means only one discern wishes a single replica of the mutated gene to bypass the increased chance of retinoblastoma directly to the youngsters. If one figure carries a mutated gene, each toddler has a 50 percentage risk of inheriting that gene.

Despite the fact that a genetic mutation will increase a toddler's threat of retinoblastoma, it does not imply that most cancers is inevitable.

Youngsters with the inherited shape of retinoblastoma have a tendency to develop the sickness at an earlier age. Hereditary retinoblastoma also tends to arise in both eyes, rather than simply one eye.

Complications

Kids handled for retinoblastoma have a risk of cancer returning in and across the dealt with eye. For this reason, your baby's medical doctor will agenda follow-up tests to test for recurrent retinoblastoma. The medical doctor may additionally layout a customised observe-up examination schedule in your toddler. In maximum instances, this will possibly contain eye exams each few months for the primary few years after retinoblastoma treatment ends.

Moreover, children with the inherited form of retinoblastoma have an elevated hazard of developing other types of cancers in any part of the body inside the years after treatment. For this reason, children with inherited retinoblastoma can also have ordinary checks to display screen for other cancers.

Preparing in your APPOINTMENT

Begin by using making an appointment together with your baby's doctor or pediatrician if your baby has any signs and symptoms or signs that worry you. If your toddler is thought to have an eye fixed problem, you'll be cited a physician who specializes in treating eye sicknesses (ophthalmologist).

Due to the fact appointments may be quick, and due to the fact there may be often quite a few ground to cover, it's a very good concept to be properly organized. Here's some information that will help you get prepared, and what to expect out of your infant's doctor.

What you could do

Be aware of any pre-appointment restrictions. On the time you're making the appointment, make certain to ask if there's something you want to do in advance, which includes limit your infant's food regimen.

Write down any signs your toddler is experiencing, together with any that may seem unrelated to the purpose for which you scheduled the appointment.

Write down key private records, such as any principal stresses or recent changes for your child's lifestyles.

Make a list of all medications, nutrients or dietary supplements your toddler is taking.

Take a family member or friend alongside. Occasionally it can be hard to recall the data provided during an appointment. A person who accompanies you may keep in mind something which you neglected or forgot.

Your time with your baby's doctor is confined, so making ready a listing of questions in advance of time let you make the most of the time. List your questions from maximum essential to least crucial in case time runs out. For retinoblastoma, some primary inquiries to ask your baby's medical doctor encompass:

What types of checks does my infant want?

What is the first-class direction of motion?

What are the options to the number one method which you're suggesting?

Should my infant see a consultant? What is going to that value, and could my insurance cover it?

Further to the questions that you've prepared to invite your baby's medical doctor, do not hesitate to ask other questions in the course of your appointment.

What to anticipate from your infant's medical doctor

Your infant's doctor is in all likelihood to invite you some of questions. Being equipped to reply them may additionally allow more time to cowl other factors. Your infant's health practitioner may ask:

Whilst did your infant start experiencing signs and symptoms?

Have your child's signs and symptoms been continuous or occasional?

How extreme are your baby's signs and symptoms?

What, if anything, appears to enhance your toddler's signs?

What, if something, appears to worsen your toddler's signs?

Exams AND diagnosis

Exams and procedures used to diagnose retinoblastoma encompass:

Eye exam. Your eye physician will behavior an eye fixed examination to determine what is inflicting your baby's signs and symptoms and signs. For a greater thorough examination, the doctor can also advocate using anesthetics to preserve your toddler nevertheless.

Imaging assessments. Scans and different imaging tests can assist your infant's medical doctor determine whether retinoblastoma has grown to have an effect on different structures around the eye. Imaging assessments may additionally encompass ultrasound, automated tomography (CT) experiment and magnetic resonance imaging (MRI), amongst others.

Consulting with other doctors. Your toddler's physician may additionally refer you to other specialists, consisting of a health practitioner who focuses on treating cancer (oncologist), a genetic counselor or a surgeon.

Treatments AND tablets

What remedies are exceptional on your baby's retinoblastoma relies upon on the scale and location of the tumor, whether or not cancer has unfold to regions other than the attention, your baby's basic health and your very own choices. While possible, your infant's medical doctor will paintings to hold your baby's imaginative and prescient.

Chemotherapy

Chemotherapy is a drug remedy that makes use of chemical compounds to kill most cancers cells. Chemotherapy can be taken in tablet shape, or it can receive via a blood vessel. Chemotherapy pills tour all through the body to kill cancer cells.

In youngsters with retinoblastoma, chemotherapy may assist cut back a tumor so every other remedy, such as radiation therapy, cryotherapy, thermotherapy or laser therapy, may be used to deal with the remaining cancer cells. This will enhance the possibilities that your baby won't want surgical operation.

Chemotherapy can also be used to deal with retinoblastoma that has spread to tissues outside the eyeball or to other areas of the frame.

CHAPTER TWO

Radiation therapy

Radiation remedy uses high-strength beams, such as X-rays, to kill cancer cells. Two types of radiation remedy utilized in treating retinoblastoma encompass:

Internal radiation (brachytherapy). In the course of internal radiation, the remedy tool is briefly placed in or near the tumor. Inner radiation for retinoblastoma makes use of a small disk manufactured from radioactive fabric. The disk is stitched in location and left for a few days even as it slowly offers off radiation to the tumor. Putting radiation near the tumor reduces the risk that treatment will have an effect on healthy eye tissue.

External beam radiation. Outside beam radiation grants high-powered beams to the tumor from a large device outdoor of the body. As your toddler lies on a table, the gadget movements around your toddler, turning in the radiation. Outside beam radiation can motive facet results when radiation beams attain the delicate areas round the eye, such as the brain. Because of this, outside beam radiation is typically reserved for youngsters with advanced retinoblastoma and those for whom other remedies have not worked.

Laser remedy (laser photocoagulation)

All through laser therapy, a laser is used to damage blood vessels that deliver oxygen and nutrients to the tumor. With out a supply for gas, cancer cells can also die.

Cryotherapy makes use of excessive cold to kill most cancers cells. During cryotherapy, a completely cold substance, together with liquid nitrogen, is positioned in or close to the cancer cells. As soon as the cells freeze, the bloodless substance is eliminated and the cells thaw. This technique of freezing and thawing, repeated a few instances in every cryotherapy consultation, causes the cancerous cells to die.

Warmth remedies (thermotherapy)

Thermotherapy makes use of excessive warmness to kill most cancers cells. All through thermotherapy, heat is directed at the cancer cells using ultrasound, microwaves or lasers.

Whilst the tumor is too massive to be handled via other techniques, surgical procedure can be used to treat retinoblastoma. In those situations, surgical operation to do away with the attention may additionally help prevent the spread of most cancers to other elements of the frame. Surgical treatment for retinoblastoma consists of:

Surgical operation to remove the affected eye (enucleation). During surgical procedure to put off the eye, surgeons disconnect the muscle groups and tissue around the eye and eliminate the eyeball. A part of the optic nerve, which extends from the back of the eye into the brain, also is removed.

Surgical operation to place an eye implant. Without delay after the eyeball is eliminated, the health care professional places a unique ball made from plastic or other materials in the eye socket. The muscle groups that control eye movement are connected to the implant. After your child heals, the eye muscle tissue will adapt to the implanted eyeball, so it can move simply because the natural eye did. However, the implanted eyeball cannot see.

Becoming an artificial eye. Several weeks after surgical procedure, a custom-made synthetic eye can be positioned over the eye implant. The artificial eye may be made to healthy your infant's healthy eye. The artificial eye sits at the back of the eyelids and clips onto the attention implant. As your child's eye muscle tissue move the eye implant, it's going to seem that your child is transferring the synthetic eye.

Facet results of surgery encompass infection and bleeding. Eliminating an eye will have an effect on your toddler's imaginative and prescient, though most children will adapt to the loss of an eye fixed through the years.

Medical trials

Medical trials are studies to test new remedies and new methods of the usage of present remedies. Even as medical trials provide your infant a danger to try the present day in retinoblastoma treatments, they cannot guarantee a cure. Ask your infant's health practitioner whether or not your child is eligible to participate in scientific trials. Your toddler's medical doctor can speak the advantages and risks of enrolling in a medical trial.

In most instances, medical doctors are not sure what causes retinoblastoma, so there's no established manner to save you the sickness.

Prevention for families with inherited retinoblastoma

In households with the inherited form of retinoblastoma, preventing retinoblastoma may not be viable. However, genetic checking out enables households to recognize which kids have an improved hazard of retinoblastoma, so eye exams can start at an early age. That way, retinoblastoma may be diagnosed very early whilst the tumor is small and a risk for a therapy and preservation of vision is still viable.

In case your health practitioner determines that your child's retinoblastoma become resulting from an inherited genetic mutation, your circle of relatives can be noted a genetic counselor.

Your child with retinoblastoma is vulnerable to other related cancers

Your other youngsters are susceptible to retinoblastoma and other associated cancers, so that they can start eye checks at an early age

You and your associate have the opportunity of passing the genetic mutation on to future kids

The genetic counselor can discuss the dangers and advantages of genetic testing and help you make a decision whether you, your accomplice or your different kids could be tested for the genetic mutation.

COPING AND assist

When your baby is recognized with most cancers, it's not unusual to feel a range of feelings from surprise and disbelief to guilt and anger. Absolutely everyone unearths his or her very own manner of handling traumatic situations, however in case you're feeling misplaced, you may try to:

Accumulate all the information you need. Discover enough approximately retinoblastoma to sense cozy making decisions approximately your toddler's care. Communicate with your child's health care crew. Hold a listing of inquiries to ask at the subsequent appointment. Go to your nearby library and ask for help looking for data.

Consult the web sites of the national most cancers Institute and the american cancer Society for extra statistics.

Arrange a assist network. Find pals and own family who can help aid you as a caregiver. Loved ones can accompany your child to health practitioner visits or sit down through his or her bedside in the health facility whilst you can not be there. Whilst you're together with your baby, your pals and own family can help out via spending time along with your other youngsters or assisting around your property.

Take benefit of sources for children with most cancers. Are seeking for out special assets for households of youngsters with most cancers. Ask your health facility's social employees about what's available. Aid organizations for mother and father and siblings put you in contact with folks who recognize what you feel. Your own family can be eligible for summer time camps, transient housing and different help.

Hold normalcy as a whole lot as viable. Small youngsters can not understand what is taking place to them as they go through cancer remedy. To help your baby cope, try and maintain a normal recurring as tons as feasible.

Attempt to set up appointments so that your baby can have a set nap time each day. Have routine mealtimes. Allow time for play when your toddler feels up to it. In case your child must spend time in the health facility, bring gadgets from domestic that allows her or him experience more at ease.

Ask your fitness care team approximately other methods to consolation your baby via his or her treatment. Some hospitals have endeavor therapists or toddler-life workers who can come up with greater precise methods to help your toddler to cope.

THE END